5 Ingredient Mediterranean

33 Easy & Amazing Recipes for Unforgettable Flavorful Feasts

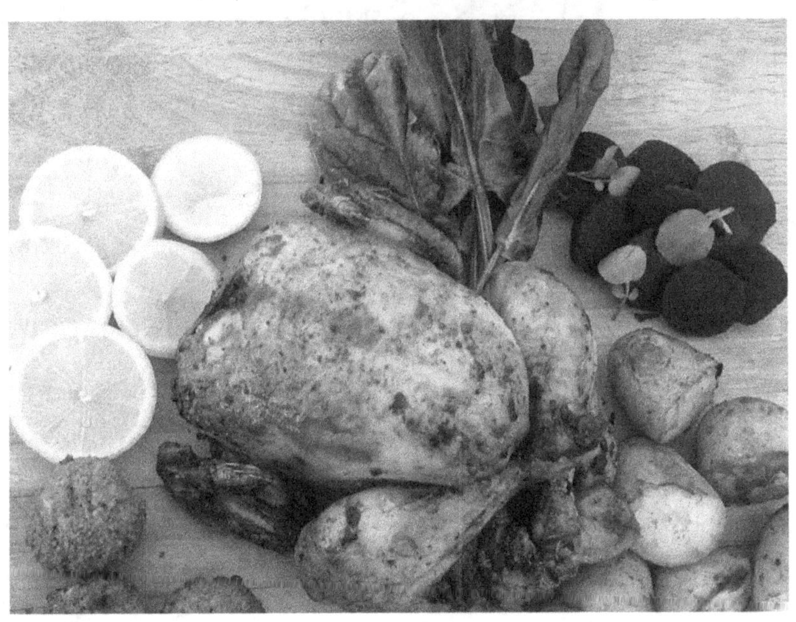

Benedict Robinson

TABLE OF CONTENTS

How to Cook Mediterranean Food with These 5 Ingredients

There has never been a more delicious or effortless way to go on a Mediterranean gastronomic trip. With just five basic ingredients at the center of each recipe, this cookbook is made to easily and quickly bring the colorful tastes of the Mediterranean to your table. Here are five quick steps to help you get started and maximize the contents of your 5 Ingredient Mediterranean cookbook:

Step 1: Embrace the Mediterranean Staples
Begin by becoming acquainted with the five heroes of this cookbook: olive oil for cooking, extra virgin olive oil for dressing and finishing meals, red wine vinegar for its flexible acidity, and the necessary seasonings of sea salt and black pepper. These ingredients are the foundation of Mediterranean cuisine and will be your constant companions on this gastronomic voyage.

Step 2: Select Your Adventure
Go through the chapters, starting with Salads and ending with Desserts, and select dishes based on what you're craving, what you follow for your diet, or the occasion. Every day presents a fresh opportunity to discover Mediterranean flavors, whether your craving is for a robust lamb chop with rosemary or a light and refreshing Greek Village Salad.

Step 3: Plan and Prep
Each recipe calls for just five primary ingredients, making preparation and buying simple. Note down the fresh ingredients you'll need for the coming week.

Keep in mind that the simplicity and high quality of ingredients used in Mediterranean cooking are what make it so beautiful. Feel free to modify these recipes according to availability or personal taste as they are meant to be adaptable.

Step 4: Cook with Confidence

This cookbook's recipes are all simple, emphasizing both technique and the inherent flavors of the ingredients. When creating each dish, use the methods as a guide, but don't be afraid to add your twist. These recipes are designed to be joyful and stress-free, regardless of your level of experience in the kitchen. Look for changes and recommendations that could serve as the basis for your next recipe.

Step 5: Savor and Share

Mediterranean cooking is all about the flavors and the pleasure of sharing meals with others. Enjoy these recipes with your loved ones as a way to celebrate the health advantages of eating a Mediterranean diet and its rich tapestry of flavors. Accept the Mediterranean custom of long lunches, vibrant discussions, and the pure joy of delicious cuisine.

Keep in mind that this cookbook is an invitation to adopt a lifestyle that celebrates community, health, and simplicity rather than just recipes. Enjoy the journey, one flavorful feast at a time.

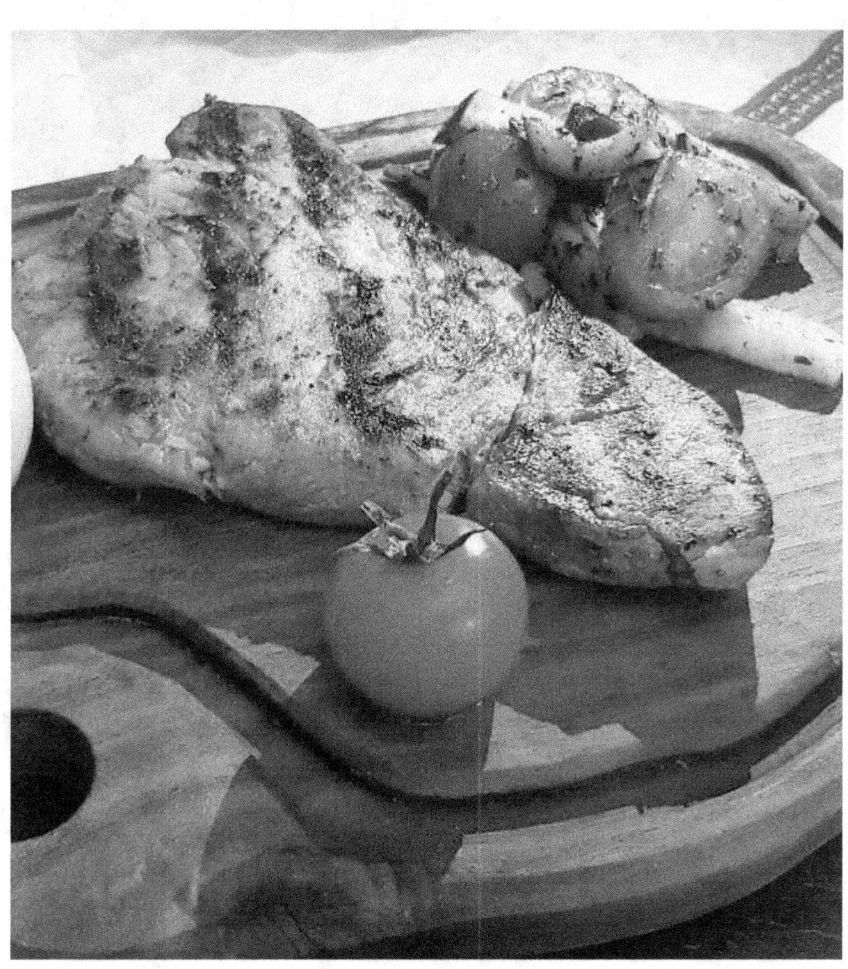

INTRODUCTION

In the heart of the Mediterranean, where the sea meets beautiful landscapes and old history whispers through the olive orchards, there is a secret to good living. It's not simply the beautiful scenery or the slow pace of life that makes this place so desirable; it's the food. Mediterranean food is simple, fresh, and unpretentiously elegant, demonstrating the beauty of high-quality ingredients combined in perfect harmony. This is the base upon which the "5 Ingredient Mediterranean" cookbook is built.

Imagine eating in a way that makes you feel like you're on a permanent vacation, with each meal celebrating flavor and wellness. That is the promise of the Mediterranean diet, which is well-known not just for its deliciousness but also for its many health benefits. According to research, this diet can boost heart health, help with weight loss, and even extend longevity. But how often do we reject the concept of fitting such a diet into our hectic lives, believing it necessitates exotic foods and hours in the kitchen?

Herein lies the secret to the "5 Ingredient Mediterranean" cookbook. It demystifies the Mediterranean diet, making it accessible to everybody, regardless of culinary talent or time constraints. With only five fundamental ingredients per recipe, this book invites you to experience the vivid tastes of the Mediterranean without the fuss. Olive oil, extra virgin olive oil, red wine vinegar, sea salt, and black pepper are the simple but transformational ingredients that may transform your kitchen into a Mediterranean oasis.

This cookbook is more than simply a collection of recipes; it's a manual for a new way of eating and living.

Each recipe is designed to bring forth the most in its components, highlighting their inherent flavors without overpowering them. From the zesty zest of a Greek Village Salad to the comforting warmth of Tomato and Basil Soup, each meal exemplifies the power of simplicity.

However, the "5 Ingredient Mediterranean" cookbook provides more than just gastronomic delights. It opens the door to a lifestyle that prioritizes balance, health, and the joy of sharing wonderful meals with loved ones. It's an invitation to slow down, enjoy each bite, and reconnect with the simple pleasures that nourish both body and soul.

So, whether you're a seasoned chef or a beginner in the kitchen, let this cookbook guide you to a better, happier way of eating. Embrace simplicity, celebrate tastes, and accompany us on a journey to the heart of Mediterranean cuisine. Welcome to the "5 Ingredient Mediterranean" cookbook, where each meal represents a step toward a more savory and satisfying existence.

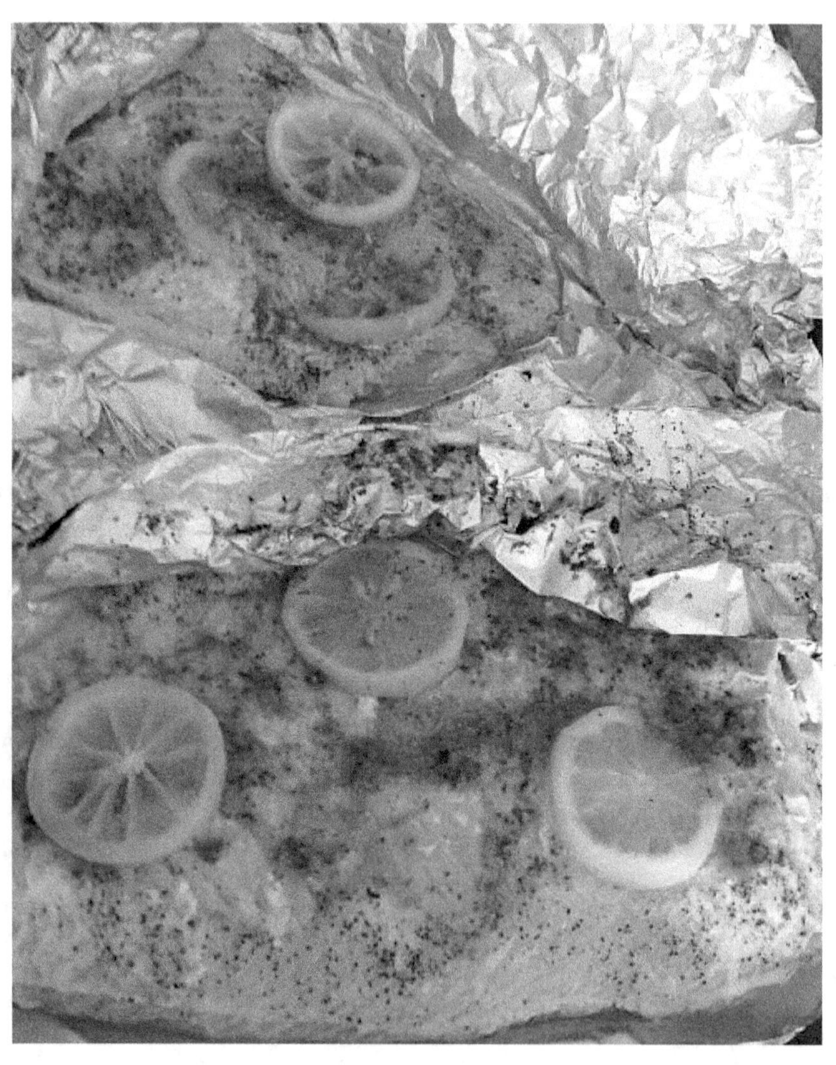

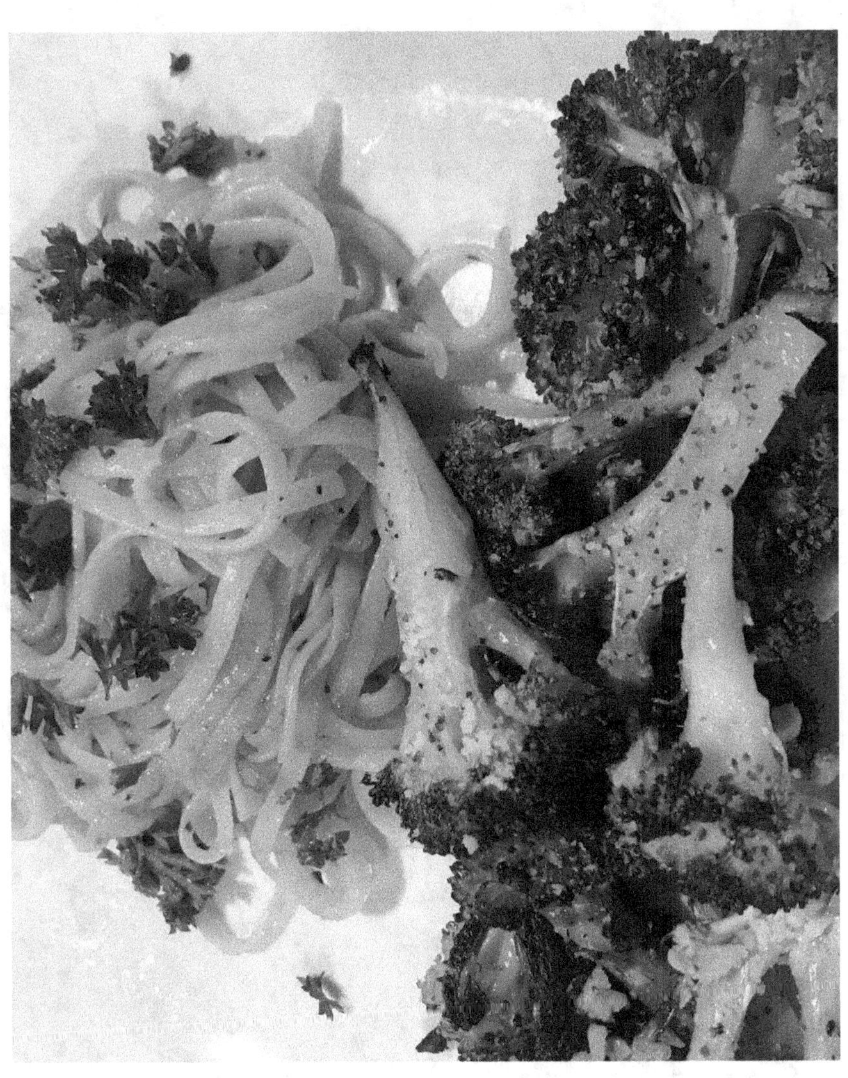

SALADS

Greek Village Salad

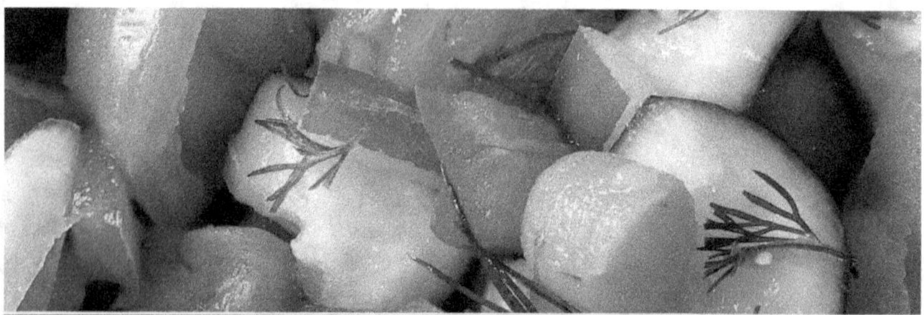

INGREDIENTS:

4 large ripe tomatoes, cut into wedges
1 cucumber, sliced into half-moons
200g (7 oz) feta cheese, crumbled or sliced
1/2 cup Kalamata olives
1/4 red onion, thinly sliced
For the Dressing:
3 tablespoons extra virgin olive oil
1 tablespoon red wine vinegar
Sea salt and black pepper to taste

METHODS:

1. Salad Ingredients: In a large bowl, combine tomatoes, cucumber, feta, olives, and onion.
2. Prepare the dressing. Mix the olive oil, red wine vinegar, salt, and pepper.
3. Dress Salad: Drizzle the dressing over the salad and gently mix. Adjust the seasoning as needed.
4. Serve: Enjoy the salad right away, offering a vibrant mix of Mediterranean flavors.

PREP TIME

10 MINUTES

Tomato and Mozzarella Salad

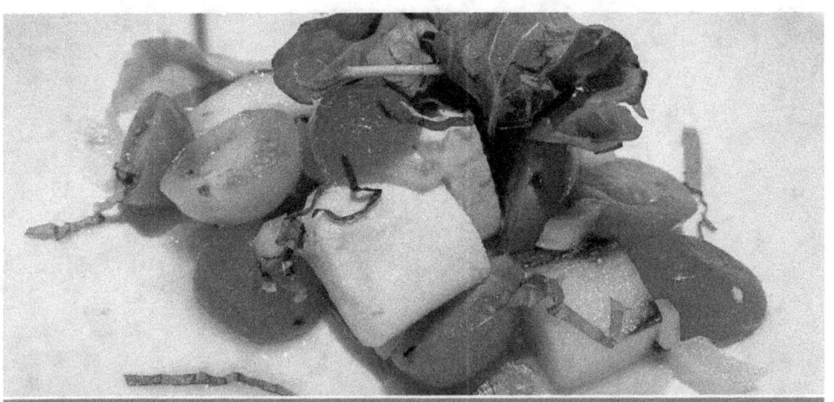

INGREDIENTS:

2 cups cherry tomatoes, halved
8 oz (225g) mozzarella balls, halved or quartered if large
1/4 cup fresh basil leaves, torn or chopped
For the Dressing:
2 tablespoons extra virgin olive oil
1 tablespoon balsamic glaze
Sea salt and black pepper to taste

METHODS:

1. Salad: In a large mixing bowl, combine halved cherry tomatoes, mozzarella balls, and fresh basil.
2. Prepare the dressing. In a small bowl or jar, combine the extra virgin olive oil and balsamic glaze. Season with sea salt and black pepper to taste.
3. Drizzle the dressing over the salad and gently mix until coated.
4. Adjust the seasoning as needed and serve the salad fresh.

PREP TIME

10 MINUTES

Cucumber and Yogurt Salad

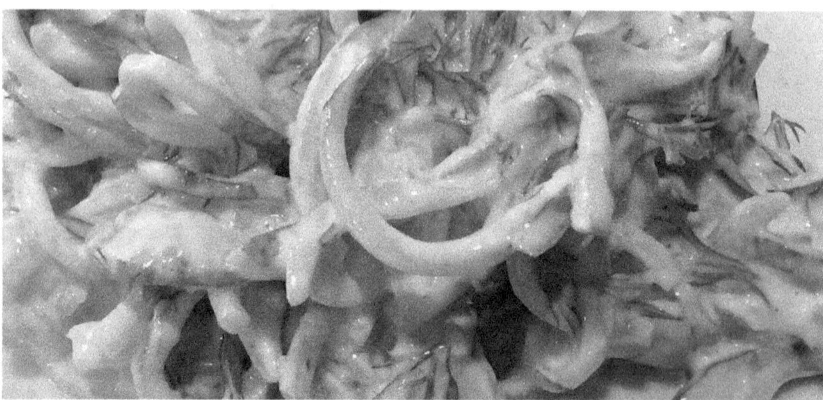

INGREDIENTS:

2 large cucumbers, diced
1 cup Greek yogurt
For the Dressing:
2 cloves garlic, minced
2 tablespoons fresh dill, chopped
1 tablespoon lemon juice
Sea salt and black pepper to taste

METHODS:

1. To prepare the cucumbers, chop them up and put them in a big salad dish.
2. Mix Dressing: Minced garlic, chopped dill, lemon juice, sea salt, and black pepper should all be combined in a small bowl.
3. Combine: Drizzle the cucumber slices with the dressing. When everything is fully combined and coated, add the Greek yogurt and stir.
4. Chill & Serve: Refrigerate the salad for 10 minutes to let the flavors meld. Serve chilled, giving it a quick stir before serving.

PREP TIME

10 MINUTES

SOUPS AND SANDWICHES

Mediterranean Lentil Soup

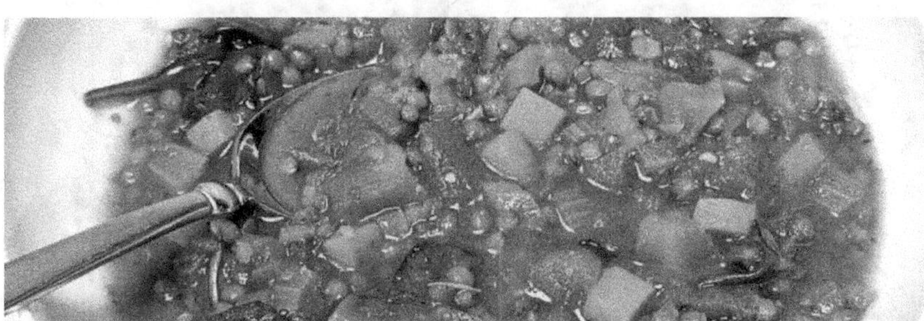

INGREDIENTS:

1 cup dried lentils, rinsed and drained
2 large carrots, diced
1 large onion, finely chopped
2 cloves garlic, minced
1 teaspoon ground cumin
4 cups vegetable broth
Sea salt and black pepper to taste

METHODS:

1. Sauté Vegetables: In a big saucepan, heat a drizzle of olive oil on medium heat.
2. Add the chopped onion, carrots, and garlic. Sauté for about 5 minutes until the onions are transparent and the carrots are softening.
3. Add lentils and seasonings. Cook for another minute, stirring in the lentils and ground cumin to combine the flavors.
4. Simmer Soup: Add the vegetable broth. Bring the mixture to a boil, then reduce the heat and simmer for 35-40 minutes, or until the lentils are cooked.
5. Season and serve the soup with sea salt and black pepper to taste. Serve hot with crusty bread, if desired.

COOKING & PREP TIME

20 MINUTES

Tomato and Basil Soup

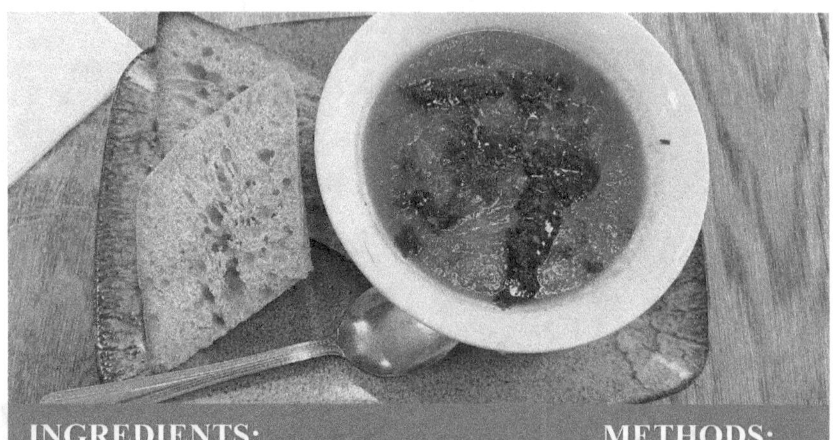

INGREDIENTS:

4 cups ripe tomatoes, chopped (or canned whole tomatoes)
1/2 cup fresh basil leaves, torn
2 cloves garlic, minced
1 small onion, chopped
4 cups vegetable broth
Sea salt and black pepper to taste

METHODS:

1. Sauté garlic and onion in olive oil over medium heat in a large pot until onion is soft (about 5 minutes).
2. Add tomatoes (with juices if using canned) and vegetable broth, then bring to a boil. Reduce to a simmer for 20 minutes.
3. Stir in fresh basil, season with sea salt and black pepper, and continue to simmer for 5 minutes.
4. Blend the soup directly in the pot with an immersion blender until smooth (optional).
5. Taste and adjust seasoning, then serve hot, garnished with basil leaves if desired.

COOKING & PREP TIME

40 MINUTES

Mediterranean Veggie Sandwich

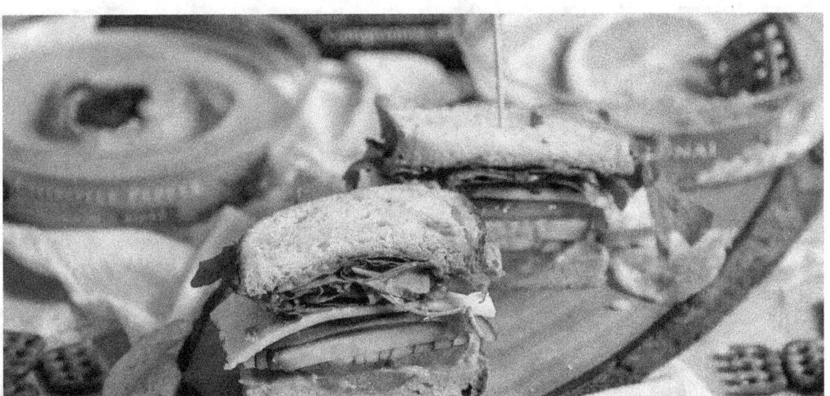

INGREDIENTS:

1 ¾ cups all-purpose flour
1 tsp baking powder
½ tsp baking soda
½ tsp salt
2 large eggs
1 cup granulated sugar
¾ cup extra virgin olive oil
1 tbsp lemon zest
¼ cup fresh lemon juice
½ cup whole milk
For Glaze (optional): 1 cup powdered sugar, 2 tbsp lemon juice

METHODS:

Prep: Preheat oven to 350°F (175°C). Grease and line a 9-inch cake pan.

Dry Ingredients: Whisk flour, baking powder, baking soda, and salt in a bowl.

Wet Mix: Beat eggs and sugar until frothy. Gradually add olive oil, then lemon zest and juice.

Combine: Alternately mix in dry ingredients and milk to the egg mixture, starting and ending with dry. Mix until just combined.

Bake: Pour into the pan, bake for 45 minutes, or until a toothpick comes out clean.

Cool & Glaze: Cool 10 mins, remove, then cool completely. For glaze, mix powdered sugar and lemon juice, drizzle over cake.

Serve: Enjoy as is or with whipped cream/berries.

COOKING & PREP TIME

20 MINUTES

Simple Mediterranean Soup

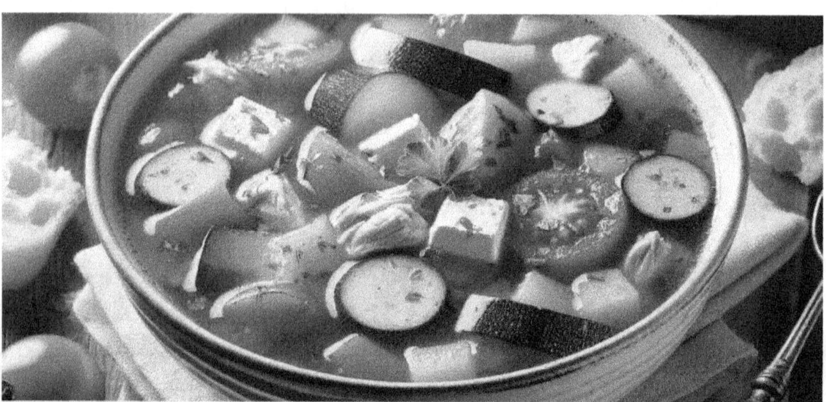

INGREDIENTS:

Ingredients:
1 tablespoon olive oil
1 medium onion, chopped
2 garlic cloves, minced
1 large carrot, diced
1 zucchini, diced
4 cups vegetable broth
1 can (14 oz) diced tomatoes, undrained
1 teaspoon dried basil
1 teaspoon dried oregano
Salt and pepper to taste
1 cup cooked chickpeas

METHODS:

1. Sauté vegetables: Heat olive oil in a large pot over medium. Add onion and garlic, cooking for 3 minutes until softened. Add carrot and zucchini, cooking for another 5 minutes.
2. Add liquids and seasonings: Pour in diced tomatoes with juice and vegetable broth. Stir in dried basil, oregano, salt, and pepper.
3. Simmer: Bring to a boil, then lower heat and simmer for 10 minutes or until vegetables are tender.
4. Incorporate chickpeas: Add cooked chickpeas and simmer for an additional 5 minutes.
5. Finalize: Adjust seasoning as needed and serve hot.

COOKING & PREP TIME

20 MINUTES

PASTA

Lemon Garlic Spaghetti

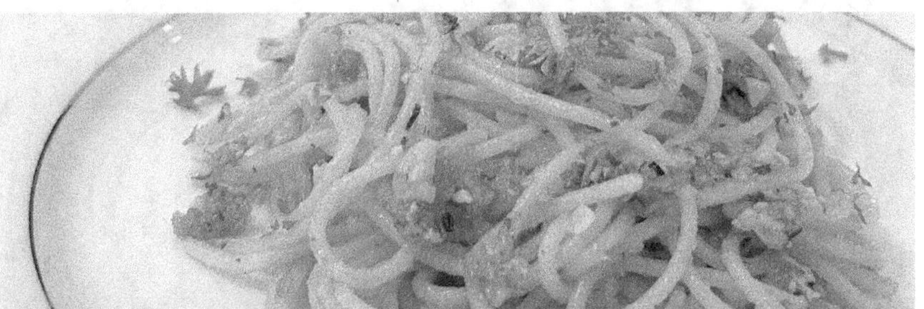

INGREDIENTS:

400g (14 oz) spaghetti
2 tablespoons olive oil
4 garlic cloves, minced
Zest of 1 large lemon
Juice of 1 large lemon
1/4 cup freshly grated Parmesan cheese
Salt and pepper to taste
Fresh parsley, chopped (for garnish)
For the Dressing:
1/3 cup extra virgin olive oil
2 tablespoons fresh lemon juice
1 teaspoon lemon zest
2 garlic cloves, minced
Salt and pepper to taste

METHODS:

1. Cook Spaghetti: Boil spaghetti in salted water according to package directions until al dente. Drain, saving 1 cup of pasta water.
2. Prepare Dressing: Whisk extra virgin olive oil, lemon juice, zest, minced garlic, salt, and pepper in a bowl. Set aside.
3. Sauté Garlic: Heat 2 tablespoons olive oil in a skillet over medium heat. Add garlic and cook until fragrant, about 1 minute, avoiding browning.
4. Combine: Toss cooked spaghetti and garlic in the skillet. Add dressing and mix well. Use reserved pasta water as needed to moisten.
5. Finish: Mix in lemon zest, juice, and Parmesan. Season with salt and pepper. Toss until pasta is well coated.
6. Plate spaghetti, garnished with parsley and extra Parmesan if liked.

COOKING & PREP TIME

20 MINUTES

Tomato Basil Pasta

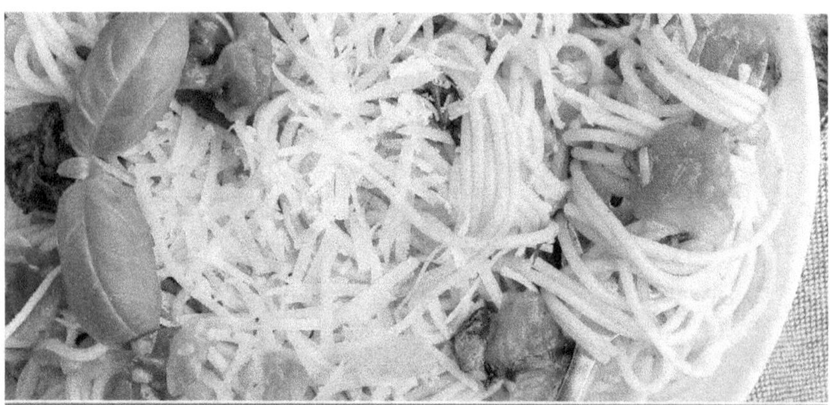

INGREDIENTS:

400g (14 oz) pasta of your choice (spaghetti, penne, or fusilli work well)
2 tablespoons olive oil
3 garlic cloves, minced
400g (14 oz) cherry tomatoes, halved
Salt and pepper to taste
1 cup fresh basil leaves, torn
1/2 cup freshly grated Parmesan cheese
For the Sauce:
1 tablespoon olive oil
2 garlic cloves, minced
400g (14 oz) canned crushed tomatoes
1 teaspoon sugar (optional, to taste)
Salt and pepper to taste

COOKING & PREP TIME

20 MINUTES

METHODS:

1. Cook Pasta: Boil pasta in salted water as per package instructions until al dente. Drain and set aside.
2. Prepare Sauce: In a pan over medium heat, warm 1 tablespoon olive oil. Sauté 2 minced garlic cloves until fragrant, about 1 minute. Stir in canned crushed tomatoes and sugar (if using),
3. Season with salt and pepper. Simmer for 10 minutes until slightly thickened.
4. Sauté Cherry Tomatoes: In another pan, heat 2 tablespoons olive oil over medium. Add cherry tomatoes and 3 minced garlic cloves, season with salt and pepper. Cook for 5 minutes until tomatoes soften.
5. Combine: Mix the tomato sauce with cooked pasta, adding pasta water or olive oil if needed for consistency.
6. Finish: Stir in torn basil leaves and sautéed cherry tomatoes. Remove from heat.
7. Serve: Plate and top with freshly grated Parmesan. Offer more cheese at the table if desired.

Spaghetti Aglio e Olio

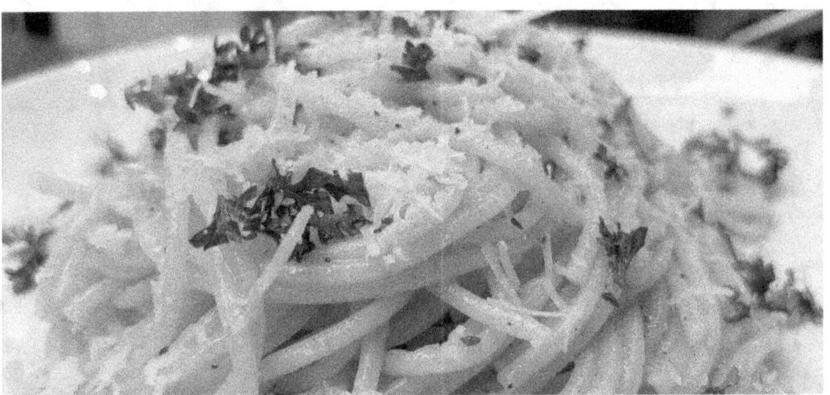

INGREDIENTS:

400g (14 oz) spaghetti
1/2 cup extra virgin olive oil
6 garlic cloves, thinly sliced
1 teaspoon red pepper flakes (adjust to taste)
Salt to taste
1/2 cup fresh parsley, finely chopped
Freshly grated Parmesan cheese, for serving (optional)

METHODS:

1. Cook Spaghetti: Boil spaghetti in salted water as per package directions until al dente. Reserve 1 cup of cooking water, then drain.
2. Sauté Garlic: Heat olive oil in a large pan over medium. Add garlic slices and red pepper flakes, cooking until garlic is golden (about 2 minutes), ensuring not to burn it.
3. Combine: Toss the drained spaghetti in the pan with the garlic oil, adding reserved pasta water as needed to moisten.
4. Finish: Off the heat, stir in chopped parsley. Season with salt to taste.
5. Serve: Plate the spaghetti, offering freshly grated Parmesan on the side if liked.

COOKING & PREP TIME

15 MINUTES

VEGETABLES

Roasted Mediterranean Vegetables

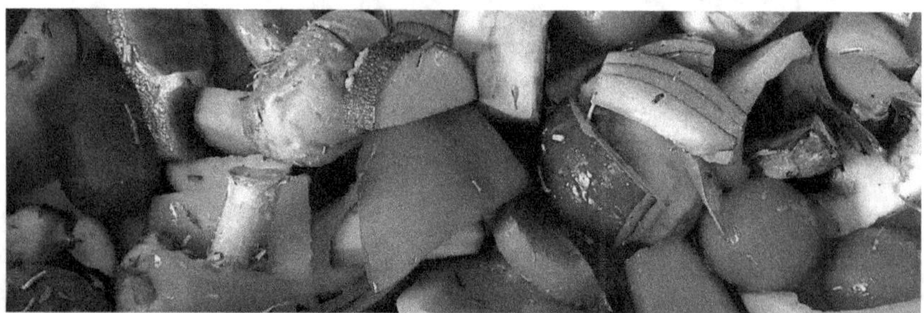

INGREDIENTS:

1 zucchini, cut into bite-sized pieces
1 yellow squash, cut into bite-sized pieces
1 red bell pepper, cut into bite-sized pieces
1 yellow bell pepper, cut into bite-sized pieces
1 red onion, cut into wedges
2 tablespoons olive oil
Salt and pepper to taste
2 teaspoons dried Italian herbs (or a mix of dried oregano, basil, and thyme)
1/2 cup cherry tomatoes, halved
Fresh basil leaves, for garnish
For the Dressing:
3 tablespoons extra virgin olive oil
1 tablespoon balsamic vinegar
1 garlic clove, minced
Salt and pepper to taste

METHODS:

1. Preheat Oven: Set oven to 220°C (425°F) and line a baking sheet with parchment paper.
2. Prepare Vegetables: In a large bowl, mix zucchini, yellow squash, bell peppers, and red onion with 2 tablespoons olive oil. Season with salt, pepper, and dried Italian herbs, then toss to coat evenly.
3. Roast: Spread vegetables in a single layer on the baking sheet. Roast for 15 minutes, then add cherry tomatoes and roast for another 10 minutes, until tender and caramelized.
4. Dressing: Whisk together extra virgin olive oil, balsamic vinegar, minced garlic, salt, and pepper in a small bowl.
5. Finish and Serve: Transfer roasted vegetables to a serving dish, drizzle with dressing, gently mix, and garnish with fresh basil leaves.

COOKING & PREP TIME

45 MINUTES

Stuffed Bell Peppers

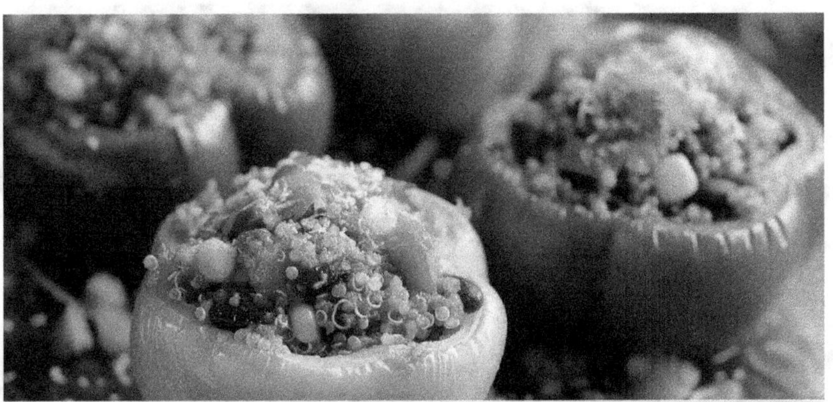

INGREDIENTS:

4 large bell peppers (any color), tops cut off and seeds removed
1 tablespoon olive oil
1 onion, finely chopped
2 garlic cloves, minced
1 cup cooked quinoa or rice
1 can (14 oz) diced tomatoes, drained
1 cup cooked black beans (rinsed if canned)
1 teaspoon cumin
1 teaspoon paprika
Salt and pepper to taste
1/2 cup shredded cheese (cheddar, mozzarella, or a blend)
Fresh parsley, chopped (for garnish)

METHODS:

1. Preheat Oven: Set to 190°C (375°F). Prepare a baking dish by arranging the cleaned and seeded bell peppers upright.
2. Sauté Vegetables: In a skillet, heat olive oil over medium. Sauté onion and garlic until they're translucent, about 5 minutes.
3. Prepare Filling: In a bowl, mix sautéed onion and garlic with cooked quinoa (or rice), diced tomatoes, black beans, cumin, paprika, salt, and pepper.
4. Stuff Peppers: Evenly fill each bell pepper with the mixture, topping each with shredded cheese.
5. Bake: Cover the dish with foil and bake for 25 minutes. Remove foil and bake for another 5 minutes until the cheese is melted and slightly browned.
6. Garnish and Serve: Let the peppers cool slightly, then garnish with parsley before serving.

COOKING & PREP TIME

50 MINUTES

Garlic Parmesan Roasted Broccoli

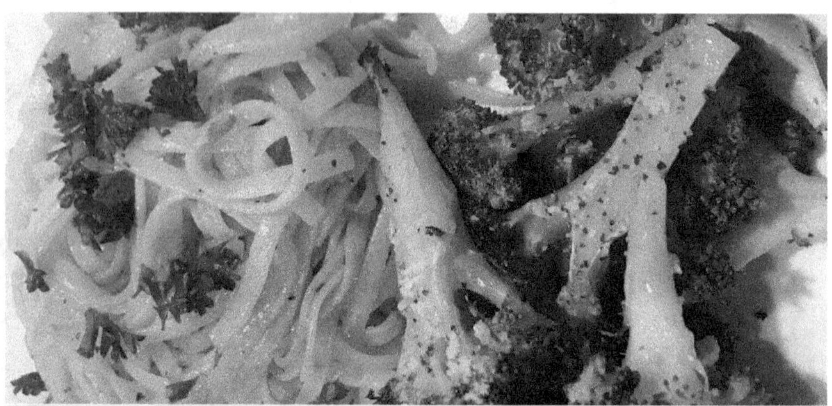

INGREDIENTS:

2 large heads of broccoli, cut into florets
4 tablespoons olive oil
4 garlic cloves, minced
Salt and pepper to taste
1/2 cup grated Parmesan cheese
Lemon wedges, for serving

METHODS:

1. Preheat Oven: Set to 220°C (425°F) and prepare a baking sheet with parchment paper.
2. Prepare Broccoli: In a large bowl, toss broccoli florets with olive oil, minced garlic, salt, and pepper until well coated.
3. Roast: Spread broccoli in a single layer on the baking sheet. Roast for 15-20 minutes, until tender and edges are crispy.
4. Add Parmesan: Sprinkle hot broccoli with Parmesan cheese immediately after removing from oven.
5. Serve: Transfer to a serving dish and accompany with lemon wedges.

COOKING & PREP TIME

30 MINUTES

PIES AND PARCELS

Spinach and Feta Filo Pie

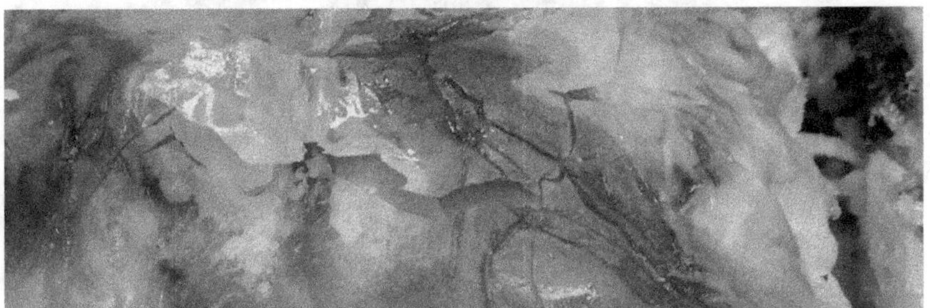

INGREDIENTS:

2 tablespoons olive oil
1 large onion, finely chopped
2 garlic cloves, minced
600g (21 oz) fresh spinach, washed and roughly chopped
200g (7 oz) feta cheese, crumbled
2 eggs, lightly beaten
Salt and pepper to taste
A pinch of nutmeg (optional)
10 sheets of filo pastry
75g (2.65 oz) unsalted butter, melted

METHODS:

1. Preheat Oven: Set to 180°C (350°F) and grease a 9-inch pie plate or baking pan.
2. Sauté Onion and Garlic: In a pan over medium heat, cook onion and garlic in olive oil until tender (about 5 minutes).
3. Cook Spinach: Gradually add spinach to the pan, stirring until wilted. Drain well, pressing to remove excess liquid.
4. Prepare Filling: Combine spinach, feta, eggs, salt, pepper, and nuteg (if using) in a bowl.
5. Assemble with Filo: Brush dish with melted butter. Layer half the filo sheets, buttering each. Spread spinach mixture over. Fold overhanging filo, then top with remaining filo sheets, 6. buttering each and tucking in edges.
7. Bake: Brush top with butter. Bake for 30 minutes until golden and crisp.
8. Serve: Let cool slightly, then slice and serve warm.

COOKING & PREP TIME

50 MINUTES

Mediterranean Vegetable Tart

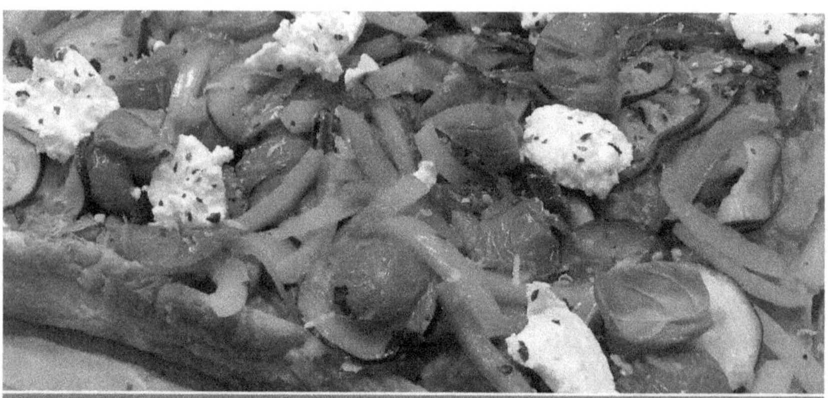

INGREDIENTS:

1 sheet of puff pastry (thawed if frozen)
1 tablespoon olive oil
1 small zucchini, thinly sliced
1 small yellow squash, thinly sliced
1 red bell pepper, thinly sliced
1 small red onion, thinly sliced
Salt and pepper to taste
2 tablespoons pesto (store-bought or homemade)
1/2 cup feta cheese, crumbled
1/2 cup cherry tomatoes, halved
Fresh basil leaves, for garnish

METHODS:

1. Preheat Oven: Set to 200°C (400°F) and prepare a baking sheet with parchment paper.
2. Prepare Puff Pastry: Roll out on baking sheet, score a 1-inch border, and prick the center with a fork.
3. Sauté Vegetables: Heat olive oil in a pan. Cook zucchini, squash, bell pepper, and onion with salt and pepper until tender (about 5 minutes). Let cool.
4. Assemble Tart: Spread pesto within the scored border of pastry. Top with cooled vegetables, sprinkle with feta and cherry tomatoes.
5. Bake: For 20-25 minutes until pastry is golden and puffed.
6. Garnish and Serve: Cool slightly, garnish with basil, slice, and serve warm or at room temperature.

COOKING & PREP TIME

40 MINUTES

Cheese and Herb Parcels

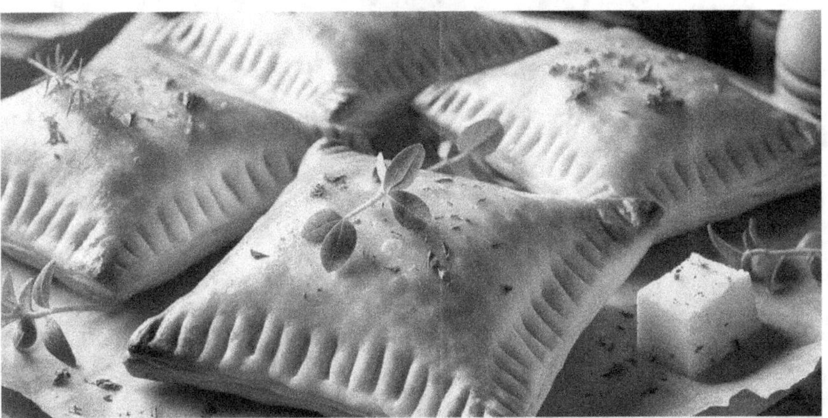

INGREDIENTS:

1 package of filo pastry (about 12 sheets)
1/2 cup unsalted butter, melted
1 cup ricotta cheese
1 cup feta cheese, crumbled
1 egg, lightly beaten
1/4 cup fresh parsley, finely chopped
1/4 cup fresh dill, finely chopped
1/4 cup fresh chives, finely chopped
Salt and pepper to taste

METHODS:

1. Preheat Oven: Set to 180°C (350°F) and prepare a tray with parchment paper.
2. Prepare Filling: Mix ricotta, feta, egg, parsley, dill, chives, salt, and pepper in a bowl.
3. Assemble Parcels: Lay a filo sheet, brush with butter, layer another on top, and brush again. Cut into squares. Spoon filling into the center, fold edges to enclose, and brush with butter.
4. Bake: Arrange parcels on the tray. Bake for 15-20 minutes until golden.
5. Serve: Cool slightly, then serve warm or at room temperature.

COOKING & PREP TIME

40 MINUTES

SEAFOOD

Garlic Shrimp

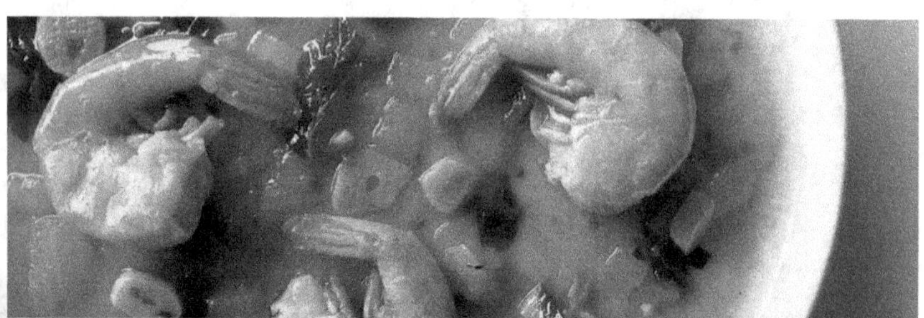

INGREDIENTS:

1 pound (450g) large shrimp, peeled and deveined
3 tablespoons olive oil
6 garlic cloves, minced
1/2 teaspoon red pepper flakes (adjust to taste)
Salt to taste
1/4 cup fresh parsley, finely chopped
Juice of 1 lemon
Additional lemon wedges for serving

METHODS:

1. Prepare Shrimp: Pat shrimp dry with paper towels to ensure proper searing.
2. Cook Garlic: In a large skillet, heat olive oil over medium heat. Sauté garlic and red pepper flakes until fragrant, about 1 minute, avoiding browning.
3. Sauté Shrimp: Increase heat to medium-high. Season shrimp with salt and cook in a single layer for 1-2 minutes per side, until pink and opaque.
4. Finish: Off heat, stir in parsley and lemon juice, tossing well.
5. Serve: Present immediately with additional lemon wedges on the side.

COOKING & PREP TIME

15 MINUTES

Baked Feta and Tomato Shrimp

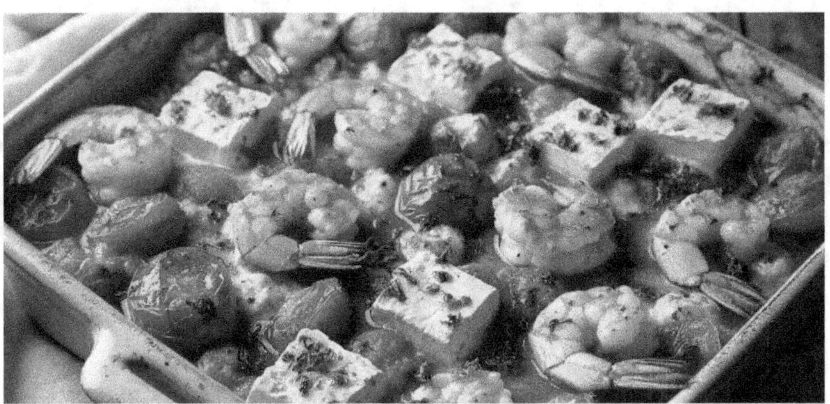

INGREDIENTS:

1 pound (450g) large shrimp, peeled and deveined
2 tablespoons olive oil, divided
Salt and pepper to taste
1 teaspoon dried oregano
2 cups cherry tomatoes
1 block (200g) feta cheese
3 garlic cloves, minced
1/2 teaspoon red pepper flakes (optional, adjust to taste)
Fresh parsley, chopped for garnish
Lemon wedges, for serving

METHODS:

1. Preheat Oven: Set to 200°C (400°F).
2. Prepare Shrimp: Mix shrimp with 1 tablespoon olive oil, salt, pepper, and oregano. Set aside.
3. Arrange Tomatoes and Feta: Place cherry tomatoes and feta cheese in a baking dish. Drizzle with remaining olive oil, add garlic, red pepper flakes, and season with salt and pepper.
4. Bake: For 15 minutes, until tomatoes start to burst and feta softens.
5. Add Shrimp: Stir tomatoes and feta gently, then nestle the shrimp in the mixture.
6. Bake Again: For 8-10 minutes, until shrimp are pink and cooked through.
7. Garnish and Serve: Sprinkle with parsley and serve with lemon wedges.

COOKING & PREP TIME

35 MINUTES

Lemon Herb Mussels

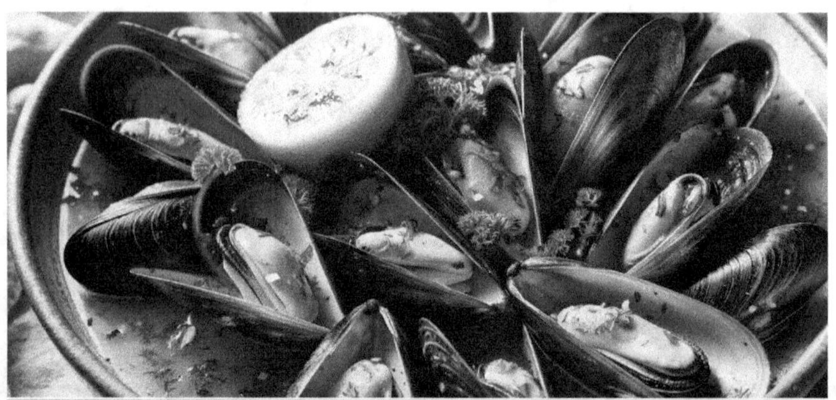

INGREDIENTS:

2 pounds (900g) fresh mussels, cleaned and debearded
2 tablespoons olive oil
4 garlic cloves, minced
1 small onion, finely chopped
1 cup dry white wine
Juice and zest of 1 lemon
1/2 cup fresh parsley, chopped
2 tablespoons fresh thyme leaves
Salt and pepper to taste
Additional lemon wedges, for serving

METHODS:

1. Clean Mussels: Rinse under cold water, scrub shells, remove beards. Discard any that won't close when tapped.
2. Sauté Garlic and Onion: Heat olive oil in a large pot over medium. Cook garlic and onion until soft and fragrant, about 3 minutes.
3. Add Wine and Mussels: Pour in white wine, bring to a simmer. Add mussels, cover, and steam 5-7 minutes until they open.
4. Season: Remove from heat. Stir in lemon juice, zest, parsley, and thyme. Season with salt and pepper. Discard unopened mussels.
5. Serve: Plate mussels with broth, accompanied by lemon wedges.

COOKING & PREP TIME

25 MINUTES

Baked Lemon Herb Salmon

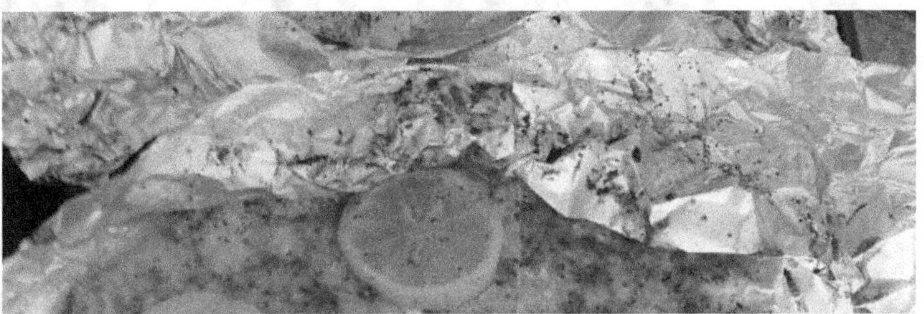

INGREDIENTS:

4 salmon fillets (about 6 ounces or 170g each)
2 tablespoons olive oil
Salt and pepper to taste
2 lemons, one sliced and one juiced
2 tablespoons fresh dill, chopped
2 tablespoons fresh parsley, chopped
1 garlic clove, minced

METHODS:

1. Preheat Oven: Set to 200°C (400°F). Prepare a baking sheet with parchment or a light oil coating.
2. Prepare Salmon: Dry salmon fillets with paper towels. Place them skin-side down on the sheet. Brush with olive oil, season with salt and pepper.
3. Add Lemon and Herbs: Drizzle lemon juice over fillets. Top with lemon slices, garlic, dill, and parsley.
4. Bake: For 15-20 minutes, until salmon is flaky. Adjust time for fillet thickness.
5. Serve: Immediately, ideally with vegetables or salad for a full meal.

COOKING & PREP TIME

30 MINUTES

Grilled Tuna Steaks

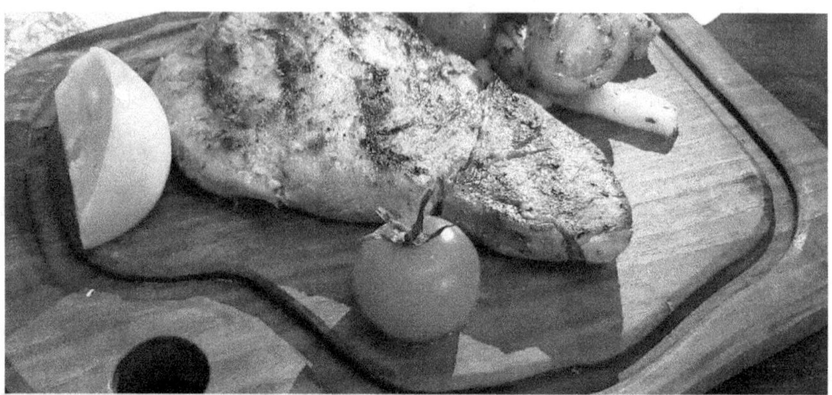

INGREDIENTS:

4 tuna steaks (about 6 ounces or 170g each, 1 inch thick)
1/4 cup olive oil
2 tablespoons soy sauce
1 tablespoon lemon juice
1 garlic clove, minced
1 teaspoon fresh ginger, grated
Salt and pepper to taste
Fresh parsley, chopped (for garnish)
Lemon wedges, for serving

METHODS:

1. Marinate Tuna: Combine olive oil, soy sauce, lemon juice, garlic, and ginger in a bowl. Season tuna with salt and pepper, place in a dish or bag, add marinade, ensuring even coating. 2. 2. Refrigerate to marinate for at least 30 minutes.
3. Preheat Grill: Heat grill to high, ensuring grates are clean and oiled.
4. Grill Tuna: Remove tuna from marinade, letting excess drip off. Grill each side for 3-4 minutes for medium-rare, or to preferred doneness.
5. Serve: Garnish tuna steaks with parsley. Serve with lemon wedges.

COOKING & PREP TIME

48 MINUTES

Herb-Crusted Cod Fish Recipe

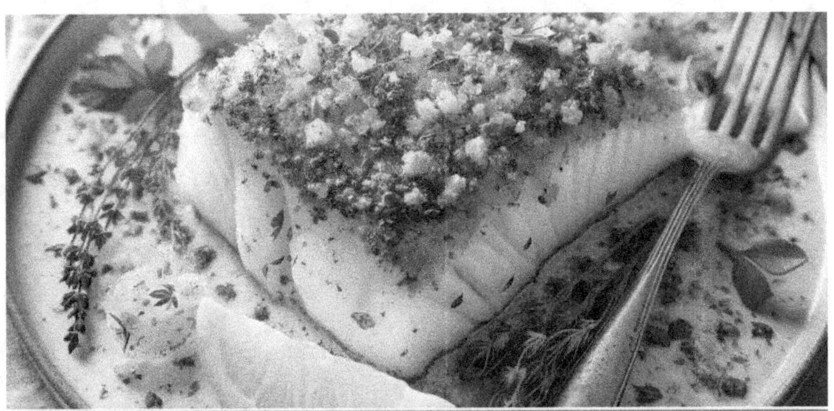

INGREDIENTS:

For the Cod:
4 cod fillets (about 6 ounces each)
2 tablespoons olive oil
Salt and freshly ground black pepper, to taste
1 cup panko breadcrumbs
2 tablespoons fresh parsley, finely chopped
1 tablespoon fresh thyme, finely chopped
2 teaspoons lemon zest
2 garlic cloves, minced
1/4 cup Parmesan cheese, grated
For the Dressing:
2 tablespoons olive oil
1 tablespoon lemon juice
1 teaspoon Dijon mustard
Salt and freshly ground black pepper, to taste

METHODS:

1. Preheat Oven: Set to 400°F (200°C) and line a baking sheet with parchment.
2. Prepare Cod: Dry cod with paper towels, season with salt and pepper, and brush with olive oil.
3. Make Herb Crust: Mix panko, parsley, thyme, lemon zest, garlic, and Parmesan with salt and pepper in a bowl.
4. Apply Crust: Firmly press breadcrumb mixture onto the top of each cod fillet.
5. Bake: Place fillets on baking sheet, bake for 12-15 minutes until fish flakes easily and crust is golden.
6. Prepare Dressing: Whisk olive oil, lemon juice, Dijon mustard, salt, and pepper in a bowl. Adjust seasoning.
7. Serve: Let fish rest briefly, then drizzle with dressing before serving.

COOKING & PREP TIME

30 MINUTES

CHICKEN AND DUCK

Herb Roasted Chicken

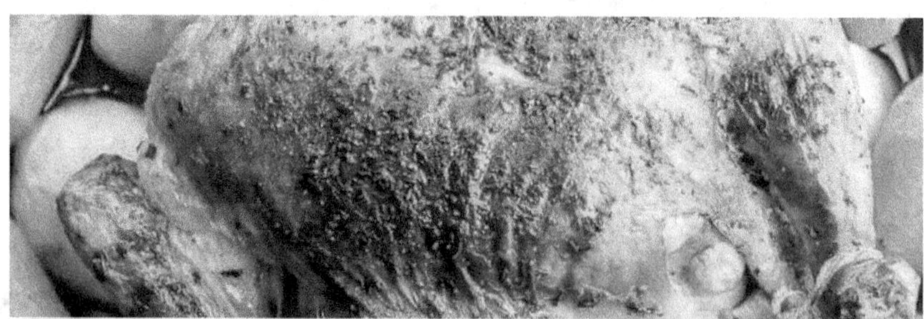

INGREDIENTS:

For the Chicken:
1 whole chicken (about 4 to 5 pounds)
2 tablespoons olive oil
Salt and freshly ground black pepper, to taste
1 lemon, halved
4 garlic cloves, smashed
1 onion, quartered
2 sprigs rosemary
4 sprigs thyme
2 sprigs parsley
For the Dressing (optional):
2 tablespoons olive oil
1 tablespoon lemon juice
1 teaspoon honey
Salt and freshly ground black pepper, to taste

METHODS:

1. Preheat Oven: Set to 375°F (190°C).
2. Prepare Chicken: Remove giblets, dry chicken with paper towels. Rub with olive oil, season with salt and pepper. Stuff cavity with lemon, garlic, onion, rosemary, thyme, and parsley.
3. Roast Chicken: Place breast-side up in a roasting pan. Roast for about 1 hour and 15 minutes, or until an internal thermometer reaches 165°F.
4. Prepare Dressing: Whisk together olive oil, lemon juice, honey, salt, and pepper.
5. Rest and Serve: Let chicken rest for 10 minutes post-oven. Serve with optional dressing drizzled over.

COOKING & PREP TIME

95 MINUTES

Roasted Duck

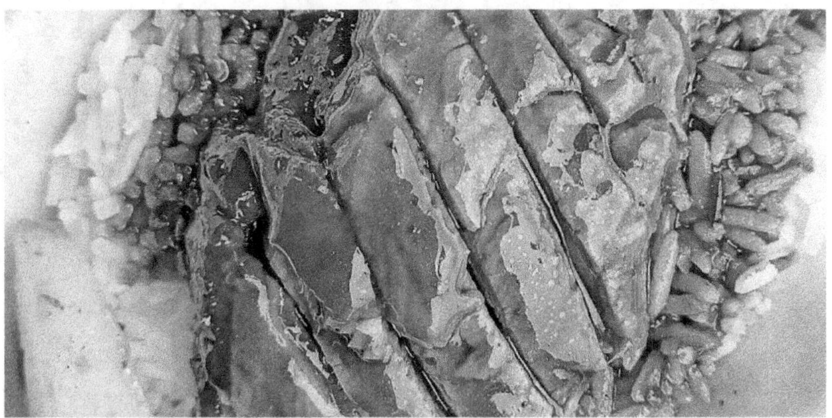

INGREDIENTS:

For the Duck:
1 whole duck (about 5 to 6 pounds)
Salt and freshly ground black pepper, to taste
1 orange, quartered
1 apple, quartered
2 sprigs rosemary
3 sprigs thyme
For the Glaze:
1/4 cup honey
1/4 cup soy sauce
1 tablespoon orange zest
2 tablespoons orange juice

COOKING & PREP TIME

150 MINUTES

METHODS:

1. Preheat Oven: Set to 350°F (175°C).
2. Prepare Duck: Dry the duck with paper towels inside and out. Score skin in a diamond pattern without cutting the meat. Season with salt and pepper. Stuff with orange, apple, rosemary, and thyme.
3. Roast Duck: Place breast side up on a rack in a roasting pan. Roast for 1 hour.
4. Make Glaze: Combine honey, soy sauce, orange zest, and juice in a saucepan over medium heat. Simmer until honey dissolves.
5. Glaze Duck: After roasting for 1 hour, brush duck with glaze. Continue roasting for another hour, until skin is browned and crisp, and internal temperature reaches 165°F (74°C).
6. Rest and Serve: Let duck rest for 10 minutes. Carve and serve with extra glaze.

Mediterranean Chicken Skewers

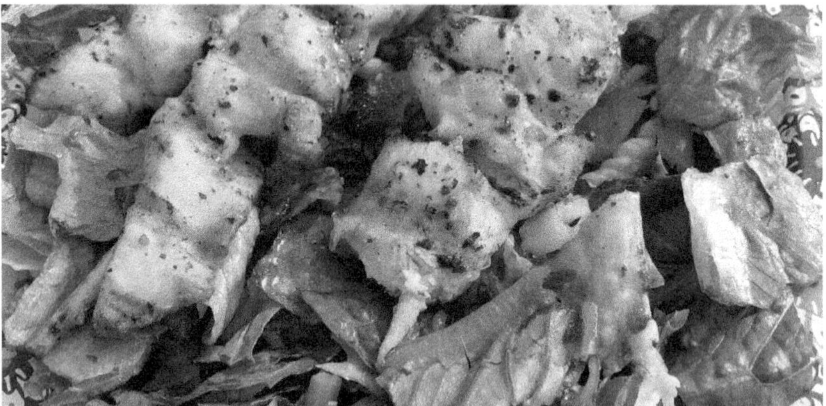

INGREDIENTS:

For the Skewers:
2 pounds chicken breast, cut into 1-inch cubes
2 tablespoons olive oil
1 teaspoon salt
½ teaspoon black pepper
2 garlic cloves, minced
1 teaspoon dried oregano
1 teaspoon paprika
1 red bell pepper, cut into 1-inch pieces
1 yellow bell pepper, cut into 1-inch pieces
1 zucchini, sliced into ½-inch thick rounds
1 red onion, cut into wedges
For the Dressing:
¼ cup olive oil
2 tablespoons lemon juice
1 teaspoon Dijon mustard
1 teaspoon honey
Salt and pepper to taste
1 tablespoon chopped fresh parsley

COOKING & PREP TIME

35 MINUTES

METHODS:

1. Marinate Chicken: Mix chicken cubes with olive oil, salt, pepper, garlic, oregano, and paprika in a large bowl. Ensure even coating. Refrigerate for at least 1 hour, or overnight for best results.
2. Preheat Grill: Set to medium-high heat.
3. Assemble Skewers: Thread chicken, bell peppers, zucchini, and onion onto skewers, alternating between them.
4. Grill Skewers: Place on the grill, cooking for 10-15 minutes, turning regularly, until chicken is cooked through and vegetables are tender and charred.
5. Prepare Dressing: Whisk together olive oil, lemon juice, Dijon mustard, honey, salt, and pepper. Stir in parsley.
6. Serve: Drizzle dressing over skewers before serving.

Mediterranean Duck Skewers

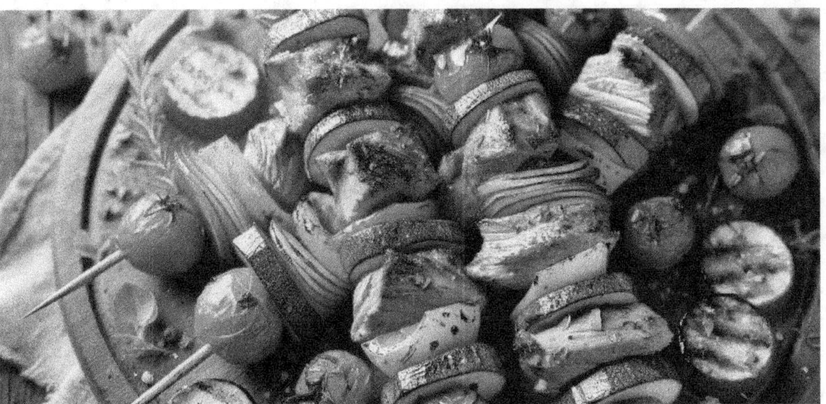

INGREDIENTS:

For the Skewers:
2 pounds duck breast, cut into 1-inch cubes
2 tablespoons olive oil
1 teaspoon salt
½ teaspoon black pepper
2 garlic cloves, minced
1 teaspoon dried thyme
1 teaspoon ground coriander
1 orange, cut into 1-inch pieces
1 fennel bulb, cut into 1-inch pieces
1 red onion, cut into wedges
For the Dressing:
¼ cup olive oil
2 tablespoons orange juice
1 teaspoon balsamic vinegar
1 teaspoon honey
Salt and pepper to taste
1 tablespoon chopped fresh mint

METHODS:

1. Marinate Duck: In a large bowl, mix duck cubes with olive oil, salt, black pepper, garlic, thyme, and coriander. Ensure duck is evenly coated. Cover and refrigerate for at least an hour, or overnight for enhanced flavor.
2. Preheat Grill: Set grill to medium-high heat.
3. Assemble Skewers: Thread marinated duck, orange pieces, fennel, and red onion onto skewers, alternating between duck and vegetables.
4. Grill Skewers: Place skewers on the grill. Cook for 10-15 minutes, turning occasionally, until the duck is thoroughly cooked and vegetables are tender and charred.
5. Prepare Dressing: Whisk together olive oil, orange juice, balsamic vinegar, honey, salt, and pepper in a small bowl. Mix in fresh mint.
6. Serve: Drizzle the dressing over the grilled skewers just before serving.

COOKING & PREP TIME

35 MINUTES

Lemon Garlic Roasted Chicken

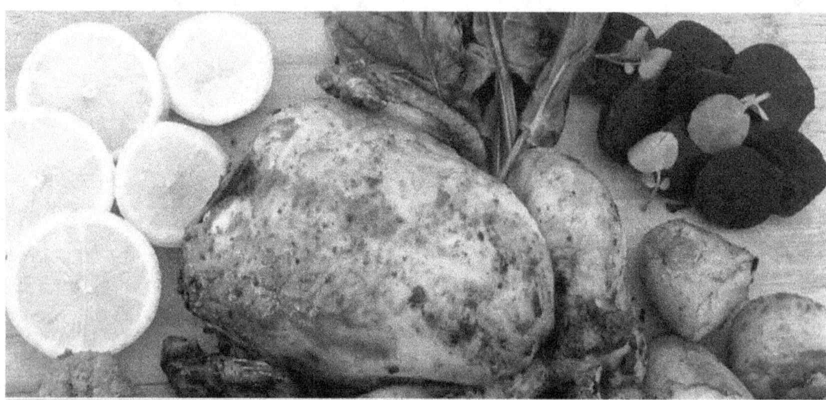

INGREDIENTS:

For the Chicken:
1 whole chicken (about 4 to 5 pounds)
4 tablespoons olive oil
4 garlic cloves, minced
2 lemons, one juiced and one sliced
1 teaspoon salt
½ teaspoon black pepper
2 sprigs of rosemary
4 sprigs of thyme

COOKING & PREP TIME

95 MINUTES

METHODS:

1. Preheat the Oven: Set to 375°F (190°C).
2. Prepare the Duck: Pat the duck breasts dry with paper towels. Score the skin of the duck in a diamond pattern to help the fat render.
3. Season the Duck: In a small bowl, mix together olive oil, minced garlic, lemon juice, salt, and pepper. Rub this mixture over both sides of the duck breasts. Arrange lemon slices and herbs on top.
4. Roast: Place the duck breasts skin-side up in a roasting pan. Insert into the oven and roast for 50 minutes to 1 hour, or until the skin is golden brown and crisp. Duck breast is best served medium-rare to medium, so aim for an internal temperature of 135°F to 145°F (57°C to 63°C) for medium-rare to medium.
5. Rest and Serve: Let the duck rest for 10 minutes before slicing. Serve with a drizzle of the pan juices enhanced with any remaining lemon juice and garnish with fresh rosemary and thyme sprigs.

MEAT

Lamb Chops with Rosemary

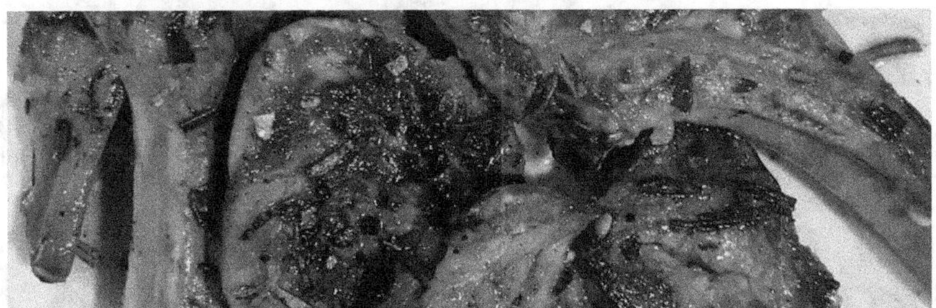

INGREDIENTS:

For the Lamb Chops:
8 lamb chops (about 1 inch thick)
2 tablespoons olive oil
2 garlic cloves, minced
2 tablespoons fresh rosemary, finely chopped
Salt and freshly ground black pepper, to taste
For the Dressing:
1/4 cup olive oil
2 tablespoons balsamic vinegar
1 teaspoon Dijon mustard
1 garlic clove, minced
Salt and freshly ground black pepper, to taste
1 tablespoon fresh rosemary, finely chopped

METHODS:

1. Marinate Lamb Chops: Mix olive oil, garlic, rosemary, salt, and pepper in a bowl. Coat lamb chops with the mixture and let marinate for 15 minutes at room temperature or up to 24 hours in the fridge.
2. Preheat Grill/Skillet: Heat grill or skillet to medium-high. If using a skillet, add a tablespoon of olive oil.
3. Cook Lamb Chops: Remove excess marinade from chops. Grill or skillet-cook each side for 3-4 minutes for medium-rare, adjusting as preferred.
4. Prepare Dressing: Whisk olive oil, balsamic vinegar, Dijon mustard, garlic, salt, pepper, and rosemary in a bowl until blended.
5. Serve: Let chops rest briefly, then drizzle with dressing before serving.

COOKING & PREP TIME

35 MINUTES

Beef Koftas with Yogurt Dressing

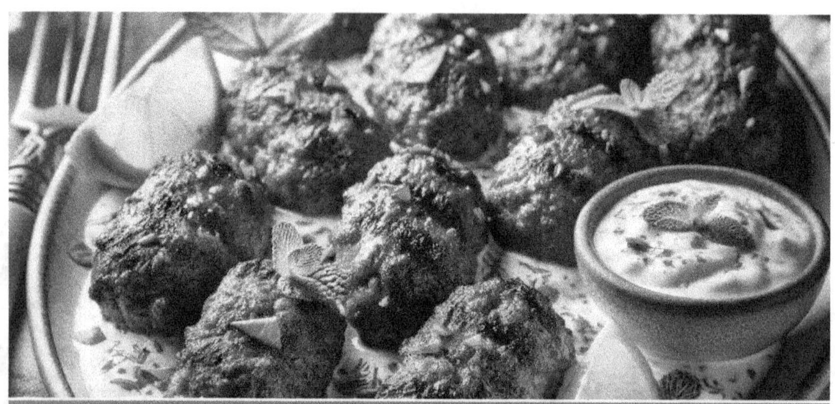

INGREDIENTS:

1 lb lean ground beef
1 small onion, finely chopped
2 minced garlic cloves
2 tbsp chopped fresh parsley
1 tsp each: ground cumin, coriander
1/2 tsp ground cinnamon
1/4 tsp cayenne pepper (adjust to taste)
Salt and black pepper to taste

Dressing:
1/2 cup Greek yogurt
1 tbsp lemon juice
1 minced garlic clove
1 tbsp chopped fresh mint
Salt and black pepper to taste

METHODS:

1. Mix Kofta Ingredients: In a bowl, combine beef, onion, garlic, parsley, spices, salt, and pepper.
2. Form Koftas: Divide and shape mixture into 8 skewers or patties.
3. Preheat Grill/Skillet: Medium-high heat; lightly oil if using a skillet.
4. Cook Koftas: Grill or pan-fry 4-5 mins per side until browned.
5. Prepare Dressing: Whisk yogurt, lemon juice, garlic, mint, salt, and pepper.
6. Serve: Cool koftas slightly, serve with yogurt dressing.

COOKING & PREP TIME

30 MINUTES

Rosemary Garlic Beef Skewers

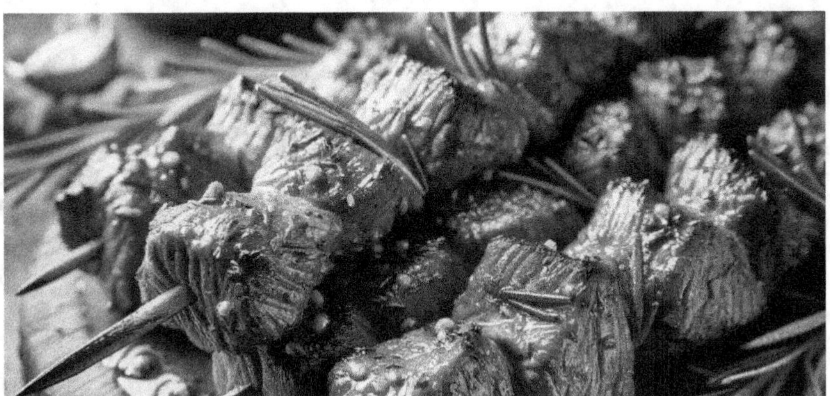

INGREDIENTS:

1 ½ lbs beef (sirloin/tenderloin), 1-inch cubes
3 tbsp olive oil
4 minced garlic cloves
2 tbsp chopped fresh rosemary
1 tsp salt
½ tsp black pepper

Dressing:
¼ cup olive oil
2 tbsp balsamic vinegar
1 tsp Dijon mustard
1 minced garlic clove
Salt and pepper
1 tbsp chopped fresh rosemary

METHODS:

1. Marinate Beef: Combine beef with olive oil, garlic, rosemary, salt, and pepper. Marinate 20 mins to 2 hrs.
2. Preheat Grill: Medium-high heat.
3. Skewer: Thread beef onto skewers.
4. Grill: 4-5 mins per side for medium-rare.
5. Dressing: Mix olive oil, vinegar, mustard, garlic, rosemary, season.
6. Serve: Rest skewers, serve with dressing.

COOKING & PREP TIME

150 MINUTES

DESSERTS

Honeyed Greek Yogurt Dessert

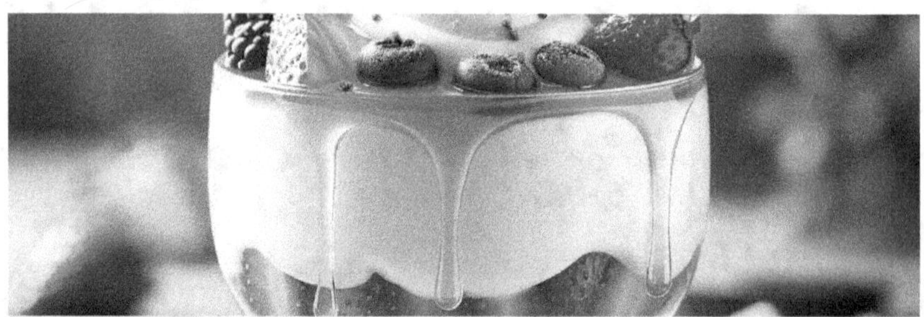

INGREDIENTS:

For the Yogurt:
2 cups Greek yogurt
4 tablespoons honey, plus extra for drizzling
1 teaspoon vanilla extract

For the Topping:
1/4 cup walnuts, chopped (or almonds, pistachios)
2 tablespoons dried fruits (such as cherries, apricots, or figs), chopped
1 teaspoon cinnamon (optional)

METHODS:

1. Mix Yogurt: Combine Greek yogurt, honey, and vanilla until smooth.
2. Prepare Toppings: Mix nuts, dried fruits, and optional cinnamon.
3. Assemble Dessert: Divide yogurt into bowls, top with nuts and fruits.
4. Finish: Drizzle additional honey on top.
5. Chill/Serve: Serve immediately or chill for a cooler dessert.

PREP TIME

10 MINUTES

Baked Figs with Honey and Yogurt

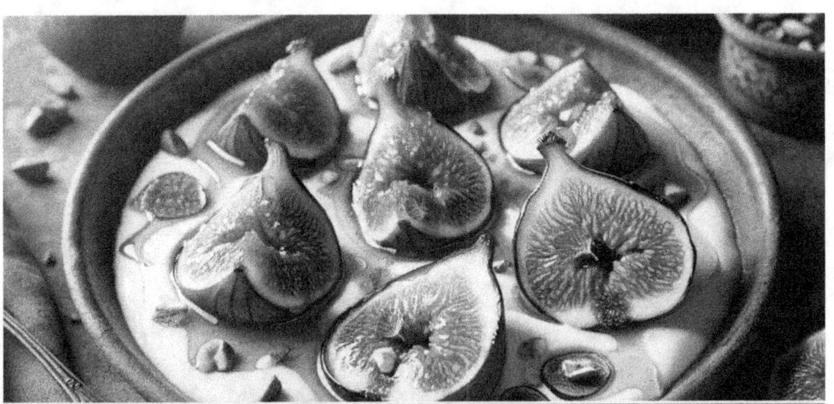

INGREDIENTS:

8 fresh figs, halved
4 tbsp honey + 1 tbsp for yogurt
1/2 tsp cinnamon, 1/4 tsp nutmeg
2 cups Greek yogurt
1/2 tsp vanilla extract
Salt, a pinch

METHODS:

1. Preheat Oven: To 350°F (175°C).
2. Prepare Figs: Arrange figs on a sheet, top with honey, spices, and salt.
3. Bake: For 15 minutes until tender.
4. Mix Yogurt: Combine yogurt with honey and vanilla.
5. Serve: Figs with a dollop of yogurt.

COOKING & PREP TIME

25 MINUTES

Lemon and Olive Oil Cake

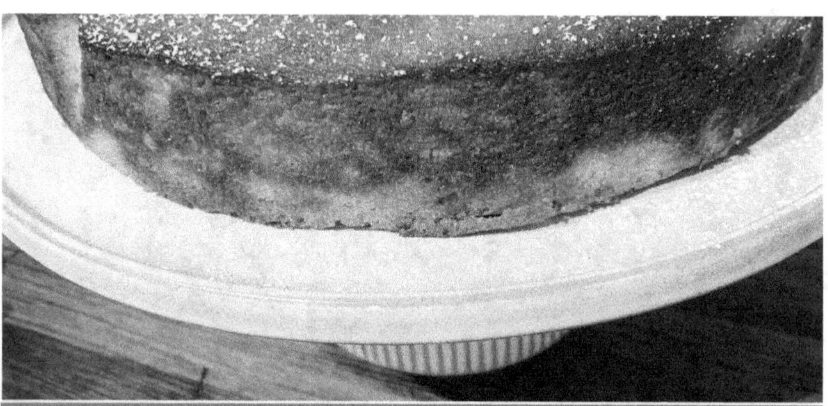

INGREDIENTS:

1 ¾ cups all-purpose flour
1 tsp baking powder
½ tsp baking soda
½ tsp salt
2 large eggs
1 cup granulated sugar
¾ cup extra virgin olive oil
1 tbsp lemon zest
¼ cup fresh lemon juice
½ cup whole milk
For Glaze (optional): 1 cup powdered sugar, 2 tbsp lemon juice

COOKING & PREP TIME

60 MINUTES

METHODS:

1. Prep: Preheat oven to 350°F (175°C). Grease and line a 9-inch cake pan.
2. Dry Ingredients: Whisk flour, baking powder, baking soda, and salt in a bowl.
3. Wet Mix: Beat eggs and sugar until frothy. Gradually add olive oil, then lemon zest and juice.
4. Combine: Alternately mix in dry ingredients and milk to the egg mixture, starting and ending with dry. Mix until just combined.
5. Bake: Pour into the pan, bake for 45 minutes, or until a toothpick comes out clean.
6. Cool & Glaze: Cool 10 mins, remove, then cool completely. For glaze, mix powdered sugar and lemon juice, drizzle over cake.
7. Serve: Enjoy as is or with whipped cream/berries.

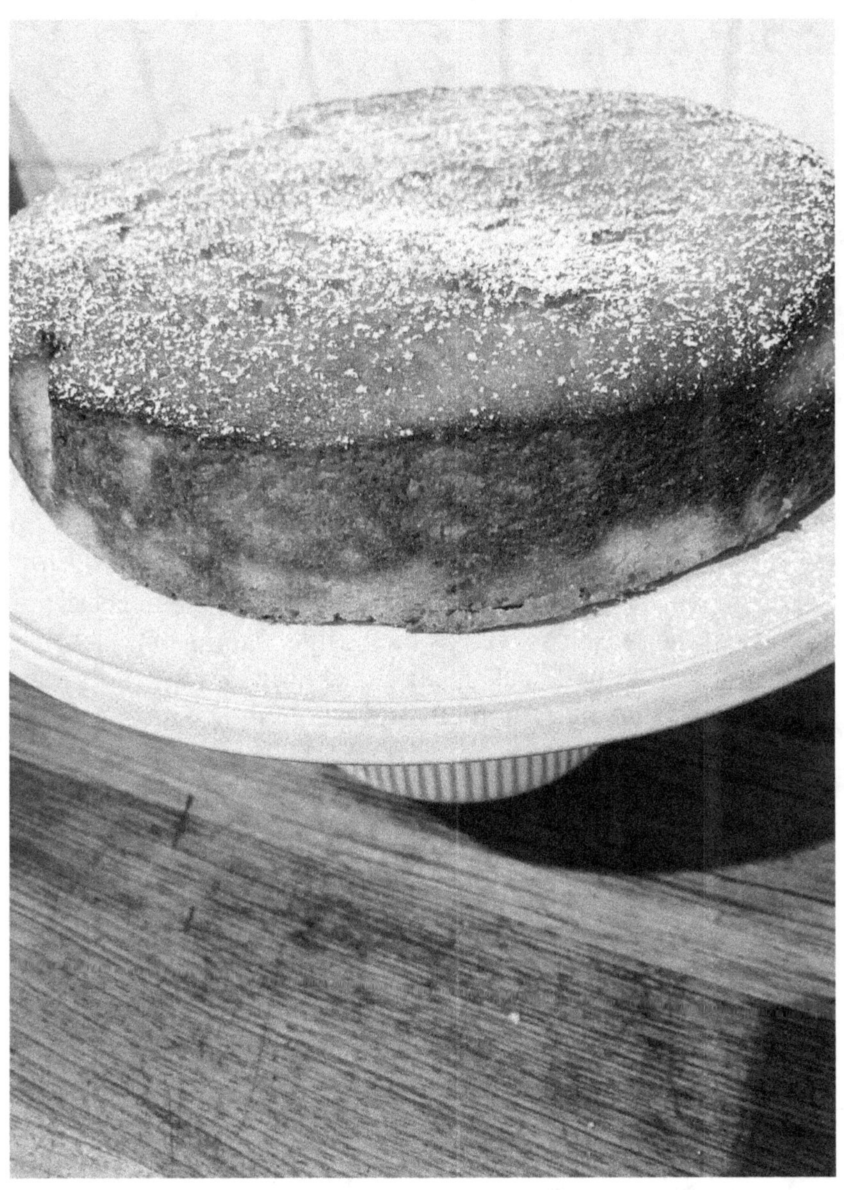

CONCLUSION

This 5-Ingredient Mediterranean Cookbook takes readers on a gastronomic journey through the vibrant and flavorful landscapes of the Mediterranean with a carefully curated selection of recipes that encapsulate the spirit of Mediterranean cuisine with the simplicity of minimum ingredients. Every dish on this page, from the delicious Lemon Garlic Roasted Chicken to the wonderful and sweet Honeyed Greek Yogurt, has been designed to gracefully and effortlessly introduce the diversity, freshness, and nutritional richness of Mediterranean food into your home.

Mediterranean cuisine is more than just food; it's a way of life that celebrates the joy of gathering around the table to share the bounty of the season as well as the health benefits of a diet rich in fruits, vegetables, lean meats, and healthy fats. You may create meals that are sumptuous and wholesome with just a few ingredients, transporting your senses to a beach that is bathed in sunlight with each bite. The goal of this cookbook is to make Mediterranean cooking easier.

As you continue to go through the recipes on these pages, keep in mind that the essence of Mediterranean cooking is flexibility and acceptance of seasonal and local ingredients. It is recommended that you adjust these recipes to your tastes, replace any ingredients that call for them, and try adding your special touch to each dish. The recipes are designed to be basic enough to inspire creativity so that you can follow the beneficial Mediterranean diet principles while incorporating your unique touches into each dish.

Rather than just adhering to a diet, when you embrace the Mediterranean diet you're appreciating food's ability to bring people together and nurture the body and the soul. Let this cookbook be the starting point of your culinary journey, where each meal is an opportunity to learn about, appreciate, and embrace the joys of leading a healthy lifestyle and where the flavorful complexity is reflected in the simplicity of the ingredients.

With this cookbook, I wish to inspire you to cook and eat with love and to embrace the Mediterranean way of life, where plenty and simplicity live in harmony. We toast to many more joyous dinners spent with loved ones and in good health in the future. Buon appetito!

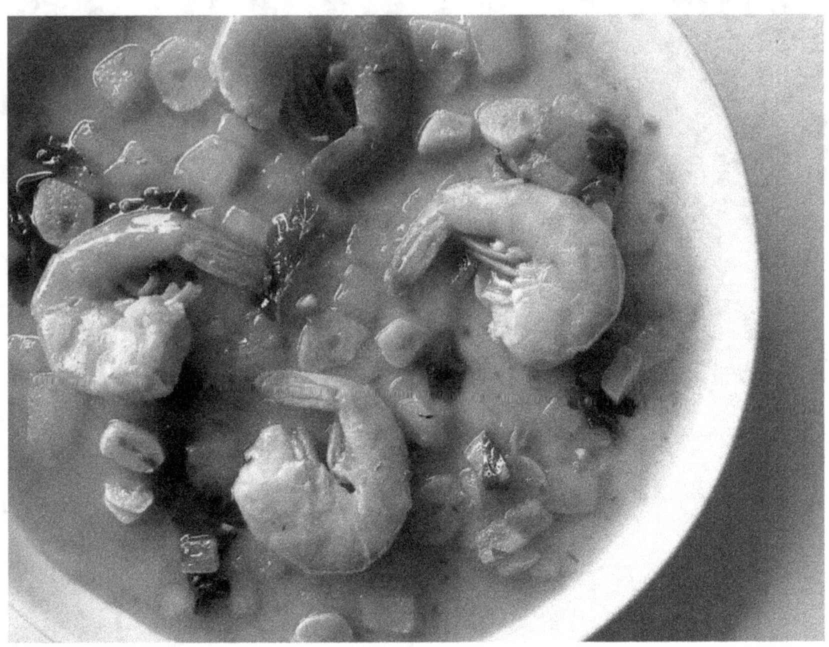

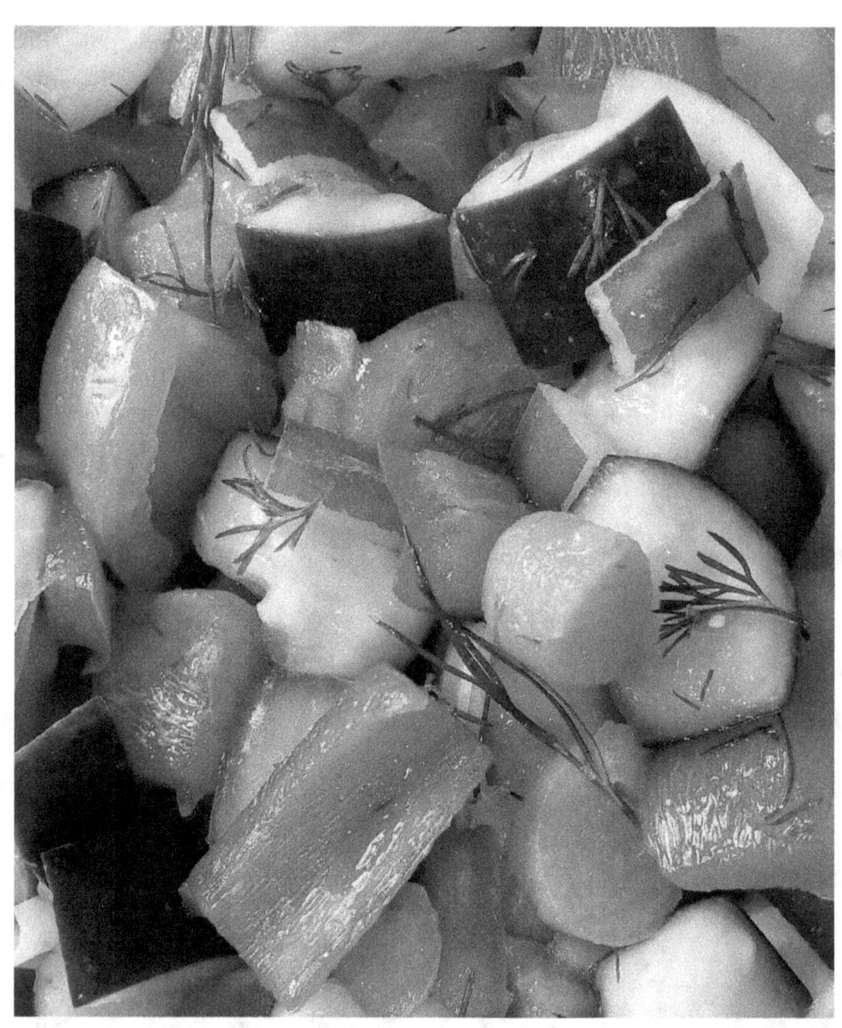

Thank-you note

Thank you for joining us as we explore the pages of the "5 Ingredient Mediterranean" cookbook. In addition to bringing the bright flavors of the Mediterranean into your kitchen, we hope each recipe has encouraged a more straightforward, happy attitude toward cooking and eating. We are delighted to offer these carefully curated recipes, whose earthy tones and complex flavors are designed to nourish the mind and body in equal measure.

As you explore the countless recipes of Mediterranean cuisine that can be made with just five ingredients, never lose sight of the fact that every meal is an opportunity to savor life's small pleasures, spend time with loved ones, and embrace the balanced, healthful way of living that the Mediterranean region is renowned for.

We are honored to share in your culinary adventures and eagerly anticipate the delectable discoveries you will make along the way. Here's to many more shared dinners, laughter, and the comforting warmth of Mediterranean hospitality. Thank you for reading, and buon appetito!